GLUTEN-FREE DIET

Gluten-Free Diet for Beginners, Including Gluten-Free Foods and Recipes

Sarah Sparrow

PUBLISHED BY:
Sarah Sparrow
Copyright © 2013

Table of Contents

CHAPTER 1: All about Gluten

What is gluten?

Gluten is an ingredient found in barley, rye and other grain species related to wheat. From the nutritional point of view, gluten is a protein composite, which means it is a protein formed from two different compounds: gliadin and glutenin. Both these components are naturally found in cereals, so gluten is a compound that naturally occurs in grains.

Gliadins represent the soluble part of gluten – but only soluble in alcohol, while glutenins are the insoluble part. The percentage of gliadins and glutenins in gluten are almost equal. Gliadins are the ones that make the dough for bread rise during baking and they're the part of gluten that the human organism is intolerant to in the medical condition called the celiac disease.

Being insoluble in water and soluble only in alcohol, gluten – and implicitly the gliadin compound, which causes the sensitivity or intolerance and triggers the celiac disease – can only be eliminated from foods containing gluten if the gluten itself is removed or if the starch that links the two components of gluten – gliadin and glutenin – is washed away.

Although responsible for the celiac disease, gluten remains an important source of protein worldwide, being a good additive to foods that are otherwise poor in these nutrients. Besides making dough rise, as already said, gluten is also used for flavoring various foods or for thickening their consistency. Outside of the culinary area, gluten – whose name comes from the Latin word "gluten", meaning "to glue" – is used for sealing envelopes, as it acts as a natural stabilizer.

Besides the already mentioned compounds, gluten also contains some other categories of proteins, but in very small amounts – less than 20%. These are called albumins and globulins and they're found in higher amounts in rice and corn.

Where is gluten found?

The first place to look for gluten is grains, these being the main natural sources of this ingredient. Wheat and products obtained from it, like wheat flour, rye, spelt, kamut, triticale, semolina, graham flour and other flours used for preparing breads and pastries, as well as the already mentioned barley contain gluten.

This much blamed ingredient is also incorporated in certain foods during the preparation process. Such products include cookies and cakes, crackers, muffins, breakfast cereals, oats, couscous, flour tortillas, pasta, gravy, various types of sauces and dressings and beer. In smaller amounts, gluten can also be found – although this isn't always the case – in soy sauce, lunch meat, soup cubes, hot dogs, croutons, rice or pasta mixes, matzo and most brands of chips.

Naturally found in grains and cereals, gluten can also be obtained or manufactured through a complex process during which grains are mixed with water, the obtained dough is left to rest so that the protein components absorb more water, then the dough is conveyed into some water tanks and washed until the starch connecting the ingredients in gluten is suspended. Once this happens, the water is forced through fine openings and all the remains are dried and then chopped into very small pieces. This is how commercial gluten results, this product being available in wet or dried form.

What is gluten used for?

Despite the numerous complaints and the negative comments on the effects of gluten, this compound remains a necessary ingredient of bread, gluten being the one that gives dough flexibility and ensures the chewy and compact composition of bread. The structure, texture and strength of bread or other pastries is strongly influenced by the presence of gluten so even if bread can still be made of oat, rice or potato flour, the composition varies greatly and bread without gluten is rarely considered "regular" bread.

How does gluten work when used for making the dough flexible and ready for baking? Proteins in this compound become flexible and longer as they absorb water and retain gases produced by yeast. The bubbles in these gases, mostly carbon dioxide, are the ones that cause the dough to expand and the bread to rise. This is one of the reasons lots of chefs use extra amounts of gluten-rich flour when they need to prepare some recipes requiring more volume or expansion, such as dinner rolls or bread loaves.

Another way gluten is used in the kitchen is as "meat imitation", mostly for vegetarian and vegan products. This is possible thanks to the "soaking" ability of gluten. Also, gluten is widely used in processed meat, thanks to its binding properties. A common compound in pizza, gluten is used for producing better quality pasta and for improving the adhesion of batter crusts to foods.

In what concerns the cosmetic use of gluten, this ingredient can be found in lipsticks, powders, foundations and body lotions, shampoos and other cosmetic products that might be threatening for celiac sufferers, according to researchers. People who suffer from celiac disease, unlike those who are gluten intolerant but aren't celiac, should try to avoid such products, as unlike foods, cosmetic products don't usually have a gluten-free label.

Is gluten good or bad?

Gluten isn't necessarily bad for your health, unless you're suffering from the previously mentioned celiac disease. This ailment is a chronic digestive condition that has very unpleasant symptoms, gluten being just as bad as poison for people dealing with this ailment.

The smallest amount of gluten can trigger an attack in such patients, which means a very serious inflammation starting in the digestive tract but affecting the entire body. The strong reaction from the organism, which has an increased sensitivity or intolerance to gluten, can damage the small intestine, causing other more or less severe health issues, from osteoporosis and infertility to intestinal cancer.

On the other hand, gluten sensitivity in non-celiac people has been traditionally considered a less severe problem, which means not all people who are slightly intolerant to this ingredient will develop an ailment that can be life-threatening.

According to The New England Journal of Medicine, there are over 55 health issues and ailments that can be triggered or exacerbated by consumption of gluten, the variety of these illnesses being impressive and worrying at the same time: canker sores, schizophrenia and multiple sclerosis can be the result or can be worsened by gluten consumption. However, as previously said, these problems are, in most of the cases, present only in people with celiac disease or gluten intolerance and the symptoms appear because their bodies can't process gluten.

But then again, the ingredient is well tolerated by a large number of people worldwide, so we can also say gluten is not threatening or harmful for one's health. So the answer to this question really depends on one's tolerance to gluten: gluten is bad for people whose bodies can't process the compound and causes no harm to those individuals who aren't affected by celiac disease or increased gluten intolerance.

According to a study taken in 2009 and 2010 and published in 2012 in the American Journal of Gastroenterology, the prevalence of the celiac disease is under 1%, which means only 1% of all people is actually intolerant to gluten and should completely avoid this ingredient. Then how comes the gluten-free diets are so popular, you might ask?

Although most people are tolerant to gluten, which means the compound doesn't put their health at risk by causing severe inflammation to the digestive tract, it doesn't necessarily mean their bodies actually get significant benefits from eating gluten-based foods.

If you want a personalized answer to the question "Is gluten good or bad?" you should try to remove all products containing gluten from your diet for one week and analyze the changes in your overall health state, energy levels, mood and digestive health.

If your energy levels are enhanced and your health state seems to improve without any apparent reason, then it means your body works very well without gluten and you can safely switch to a gluten-free diet. On the other hand, if you don't notice any improvement or your health state seems to get worse, you should maintain gluten-based products in your menu. However, statistics show for most people the removal of foods containing gluten from their diet brings benefits to their health state.

Going gluten-free doesn't necessarily mean one will eat healthier as there are lots of products that do contain gluten but also provide important nutrients, vitamins and minerals and eliminating those from one's diet can lead to nutritional deficiencies.

Is gluten addictive?

Yes, gluten can be addictive as the intake of this ingredient stimulates the production and release of certain chemicals called "exorphins", which are quite similar to the endorphins that make one happy and cause their enhanced mood. Exorphins bind to certain receptors in the brain, called opioid receptors, that are responsible for inducing a sensation of well-being and happiness and this is why the effects of these chemicals are considered similar to those caused by heroin.

The production of exorphins starts whenever proteins like gluten are digested, as the components of this compound are converted into shorter proteins or polypeptides, which are the already mentioned exorphins. These polypeptides are quickly absorbed into the bloodstream and pass easily through the blood brain barrier, triggering the specific manifestations.

While the mood enhancing effect can seem positive at first sight, it's actually a harmful one as it tells the individual that the consumption of foods containing gluten is positive and mood-enhancing. This is how the addictive eating behavior appears and this behavior is often manifested through binging and cravings for sugar and unhealthy foods.

People don't binge veggies but they do binge sugar-rich products, exactly due to these drug-like chemicals that are released into the organism when ingredients in gluten-based foods are processed and digested. This doesn't mean gluten is the worst enemy found in foods, but it's a very damaging one from this point of view, as it does take a strong will to control your cravings and say no to sugar-rich foods.

According to statistical data, as many as 75% of overweight and obese people within the United States are addicted to their carbohydrates and gluten-based products, such as bread, pastries, cookies, candies, pasta or similar foods. Unfortunately, the addiction is both biological –

caused by the chemical reactions that lead to the release of exorphins – and emotional – caused by the feelings of well-being appearing after the consumption of gluten-containing foods.

Cravings are unhealthy and problematic regardless of their cause, as they lead to emotional eating and consequently to quick weight gain. While hunger pangs signal that one is actually hungry and needs to eat food for restoring their body's energy level, cravings aren't a sign of hunger but the result of sugar and gluten addiction in most cases. And here comes the worst part: gluten is not only addictive but also highly inflammatory for people who are intolerant to this ingredient.

By causing the inflammation of the mucous membrane lining the intestinal tract, gluten forces the immune system to react and its reaction usually manifests as fatigue, tiredness, nervousness, irritability, mental fog, rashes, low energy levels,   behavioral disorders, headaches, constipation, diarrhea or other similar symptoms. How does one cope with low energy levels, anxiety, nervousness and moodiness? Obviously the easiest way is to "reward" their body with something sweet as the subconscious knows eating foods containing sugar or gluten will enhance their mood.

How much gluten is safe?

The amount of gluten-based foods one should eat depends on their attitude towards foods and on how well they can control their cravings. An individual following a rather healthy diet, who can easily keep his cravings under control and who rarely consumes sweets or products containing gluten, other than bread, shouldn't be very concerned about the amount of gluten he gets from food.

On the other hand, one who has a sweet tooth and feels the constant need of eating sugar-rich products and foods containing gluten should try to keep the amount of these products at a minimum, as even if their body tolerates the compound, addiction can still develop. This means that even if in some people gluten is "safe" from the biological point of view, as it doesn't cause intolerance symptoms or celiac disease, the ingredient remains "unsafe" from the emotional point of view, as it can cause addiction manifestations.

There isn't a standard amount of gluten-based products one should eat daily but a good strategy for avoiding the potential side effects of gluten is to stick with a diet that consists mostly of veggies, lean meat, fruits that are low in sugar, nuts and seeds and fat-free dairy products, as these are the healthiest categories of food.

Grains should also be eaten but in moderate amounts and whenever possible, in gluten-free versions. As for pastries, cookies, candies and cakes, sweet drinks and gluten-containing beverages, these can be completely eliminated from one's diet as the body doesn't really require those excess sugars and all the preservatives, additives and harmful chemicals in these products.

When does gluten become unsafe?

As said, people who suffer from celiac disease and are intolerant to gluten should completely avoid this ingredient, so in their case gluten becomes unsafe from the smallest serving. On the other hand, people who tolerate gluten well can develop sensitivity to this compound and can become intolerant in time.

The celiac disease is an autoimmune disorder, which means it develops due to a weakened immune system. But gluten sensitivity is not the same with the celiac disease (CD), although many symptoms specific for CD are also found in people who have an increased sensitivity to gluten.

Gluten sensitivity appears in people who are reactive to gluten, meaning that they don't tolerate well this compound, but their bodies don't have the autoimmune markers associated with celiac disease. Also, wheat allergy is not the same with gluten sensitivity or celiac disease: some people don't tolerate wheat-based products due to allergic reactions to other ingredients in wheat or grains, but not to gluten.

According to scientists, people suffering from celiac disease can consume up to 10 mg of gluten per day without putting their health at risk. But a regular slice of white bread contains around 3,500 mg of gluten, which is over 300 times the maximum admitted daily amount of gluten for celiac disease sufferers. So for these people, gluten becomes unsafe from the first bite.

As stated by the FDA, for the most sensitive persons, the internal damage begins at 0.4 mg of gluten per day, which is 1/200 of a teaspoon of flour! As for people who aren't gluten intolerant, don't have allergies to wheat or other products containing gluten and aren't suffering from CD, there's no daily amount considered "unsafe".

However, these people should listen to their bodies and see how they react after eating gluten-based products: are they bloated? Are headaches, fatigue and digestive problems always present after the breakfast bread serving? The "safe" dose in these cases varies from one person to another and the best thing one can do is to simply reduce the intake gradually, until they find that daily amount of gluten their bodies are comfortable with.

As for gluten incorporated in cosmetic products, this can also be threatening for celiac diseases sufferers, as these products come in contact with bodily fluids and mucous membranes and can cause unpleasant reactions.

Does gluten impact the blood sugar level?

Gluten itself doesn't have the same effects on blood sugar levels as sugar does, meaning that it doesn't cause spikes in blood sugar values and this statement has a scientific argument: gluten is a protein, and proteins – regardless of their type – only raise blood sugar slowly, which is good. On the other hand, gluten isn't eaten alone; it comes in foods that most often contain sugar or other carbohydrates as well.

Grains are rich in simple carbohydrates, while fruits and vegetables usually contain complex carbohydrates. Simple carbohydrates are quickly destroyed inside the digestive tract and glucose resulting from these nutrients is rapidly absorbed into the blood stream, causing blood glucose levels to rise. If these levels stay elevated for longer than normal, more severe health issues can appear and diabetes is just one of them.

In simpler words, even if gluten itself doesn't cause blood sugar levels to rise, foods containing gluten do, in most cases, have this effect, so if you want to make sure your glycemia remains in normal limits you'll need to completely avoid gluten as this is the simplest solution. People suffering from diabetes will experience significant improvements in their health state if they remove products containing gluten from their daily menu, as the amount of simple carbohydrates will be reduced and thus the levels of blood glucose will no longer vary so much during the day.

Does gluten interact with lactose?

While the link between gluten intolerance and diabetes or elevated blood sugar levels is quite obvious, the relationship between lactose intolerance and gluten sensitivity is more subtle and requires a more detailed explanation. Lactose intolerance is the condition in which one's body is unable to properly process milk or other dairy products that contain the compound called lactose.

Lactose is a sugar formed from two different chemical compounds, glucose and galactose. Whenever a dairy product is eaten, an enzyme is produced inside the digestive tract and this enzyme – called lactase – breaks down lactose to the previously mentioned compounds. Lactase is produced by the cells within the small intestine but when these cells don't function as they should, they can't release enough lactase therefore lactose can't be broken down to simpler sugars and metabolized properly.

What makes the cells within the small intestine unable to process lactose? These cells can have an altered functioning and structure due to genetics or can get damaged in time. Typically, the villi and microvilli of these cells catch the lactose molecules and break them down, allowing glucose to be absorbed into the blood stream. However, in people with celiac disease, these cells usually get damaged in time, so this is why people with CD are often lactose intolerant as well.

In lots of cases the symptoms of lactose intolerance disappear once CD sufferers remove gluten from their menu, as villi and microvilli of cells in the small intestine grow back and recover, thus the functioning of these cells is restored. So although gluten and lactose don't influence one another directly, eating a diet rich in gluten can lead to lactose intolerance so this is why lots of people feel bloated and accuse an overall state of malaise after eating bread, dairy, pastries and other products containing one of these two compounds.

CHAPTER 2: Gluten Sensitivity and Intolerance

What is gluten sensitivity?

Gluten sensitivity is different from the celiac disease, this term being actually used for defining a spectrum of digestive disorders, including the allergy to wheat and the celiac disease. Gluten sensitivity defines those ailments in which the intake of gluten causes adverse effects on the organism, most common symptoms being diarrhea, abdominal pain and discomfort, bloating, muscular cramps and aches, bone and joint pain.

While people with celiac disease have the cells within the small intestine damaged and this is what causes the unpleasant symptoms and intolerance to gluten, in people with gluten sensitivity these cells aren't damaged yet the body can't properly process the compound, so symptoms similar to those of CD occur.

Celiac disease appears in less than 1% of all people, as already indicated, while gluten sensitivity is a lot more common, being present in one in 10 people. However, lots of individuals are unaware of this problem and fail in linking the frequent bloating episodes, headaches or digestive discomfort with gluten intake. A gluten-free diet is recommended for people with gluten sensitivity but it's an imperative for sufferers with celiac disease. Celiac disease is diagnosed through blood tests and biopsy. These will come up positive in CD sufferers and negative in people with gluten sensitivity but who are non-celiac.

What is gluten intolerance?

As previously said, all people who have celiac disease are sensitive to gluten, this spectrum of disorders including all forms of gluten intolerance, from severe to mild ones. Gluten sensitivity manifests as mild gluten intolerance in about 15% of the US population, symptoms being quite similar to those experienced by CD sufferers.

To understand this better: both gluten intolerance and celiac disease are included in the group of ailments defined as gluten sensitivity disorders. Celiac disease is caused by gluten intolerance but there are also people who are gluten intolerant without being celiac. Gluten intolerance is not an immune reaction, while celiac disease is. This is why celiac disease can be diagnosed through blood tests that indicate the presence of certain antibodies, while in gluten intolerance these results can be negative. Gluten intolerance has a slower onset than celiac disease.

What is the celiac disease?

Celiac disease (CD) is an inherited, autoimmune disorder that starts manifesting in early childhood, as a reaction to gluten intake. Whenever people with CD eat something that contains gluten, an immune reaction is triggered and this toxic and damaging reaction alters the structure and functioning of cells within the small intestine. Once this happens, the body becomes unable to properly absorb and process foods containing gluten and unpleasant symptoms – autoimmune reactions – are caused.

Manifestations of the celiac disease appear whenever the smallest amount of gluten is eaten, which means that sufferers with this ailment should completely avoid gluten. On the other hand, people with gluten intolerance who are non-celiac can eat small amounts of gluten without having the autoimmune symptoms, although their bodies feel a lot better on a gluten-free diet.

Given that the celiac disease affects the structure of cells in the small intestine, it affects the organism's ability of absorbing all types of nutrients through the mucous membrane lining the digestive tract. As a result, malnutrition can appear even when large amounts of foods are eaten, as nutrients aren't properly absorbed inside the body. Celiac disease, also called gluten-sensitive enteropathy or gluten sprue, is genetic and runs in family.

In people with celiac disease, the immune system – which is designed to protect the organism from any type of pathogens and invaders – perceives gluten and foods containing gluten as "foreign", thus it starts producing antibodies. These antibodies are meant to protect the intestinal lining from the harmful effects of gluten, so this is why those specific CD symptoms appear.

Who develops celiac disease?

As said, celiac disease is caused by genetic mutations in a large number of people, so if you have a family history of CD, you're more likely to get the ailment than someone who doesn't have any family member affected by this disorder. However, not all people who have the gene mutations responsible for CD will actually develop the ailment, researchers say.

Theoretically, celiac disease can affect anyone with those mutations, at any time, but it can also appear in any person that eats gluten-rich foods in large amounts, as a result of a gluten intolerance that develops in time. This is why celiac disease usually stars manifesting during early childhood, before the age of 1, or in later adulthood, after the age of 40.

At higher risk of developing celiac disease or non-celiac gluten intolerance are people affected by autoimmune thyroid disease, type 1 diabetes, microscopic colitis and the Down syndrome. Also, people affected by systemic lupus, by Addison's disease, Sjogren's syndrome, rheumatoid arthritis, dermatitis herpetiformis and autoimmune hepatitis are more prone to developing CD. What's worrying is that more than 90% of all people with celiac disease remain undiagnosed, according to the Celiac Disease Foundation.

What are the symptoms of gluten sensitivity?

As previously said, gluten sensitivity refers to a spectrum of ailments, so manifestations can be slightly different for celiac disorder and non-celiac gluten sensitivity. Gluten sensitivity in non-celiac people manifests through:

- Headaches
- Joint pain
- Numbness in fingers, arms and legs
- Mental fogginess

- Muscle cramps
- Chronic fatigue

Besides these symptoms, the specific digestive manifestations of celiac disease are present in lots of cases in non-celiac people as well, but non-celiac gluten sensitivity usually manifests through nongastrointestinal symptoms. However, symptoms alone can't distinguish celiac from non-celiac gluten sensitivity, a blood test or biopsy being needed for a proper diagnosis.

Symptoms of gluten sensitivity in celiac people include gastrointestinal and nongastrointestinal manifestations. Gastrointestinal symptoms include:

- Bloating
- Gas
- Flatulence
- Abdominal distention and pain
- Constipation
- Acid reflux
- Diarrhea
- Floating stools
- Vomiting
- Nausea
- Weight variations without any apparent reason

Nongastrointestinal symptoms of gluten sensitivity in celiac sufferers include:

- General weakness
- Fatigue
- Joint and bone pain
- Headaches
- Mineral and vitamin deficiencies
- Fuzzy brain
- Depression

- Moodiness
- Irritability
- Inability to concentrate
- Eczema
- Rosacea
- Acne
- Psoriasis
- Canker sores
- Respiratory problems
- Swelling and inflammation
- Bruising
- Hair loss
- Muscle cramps
- Early onset osteoporosis
- Hypoglycemia
- Frequent nosebleeds
- Infertility
- Night blindness
- Dental enamel deficiencies
- Abnormal menstrual cycles
- Seizures
- Nerve damage
- Sjogren's syndrome
- Lupus
- Hashimoto's disease
- Lactose intolerance

What are the symptoms of celiac disease?

Symptoms of celiac disease are pretty much the same with manifestations of all disorders caused by gluten intolerance. In children, most common symptoms of celiac disease include:

- Abdominal bloating and pain
- Altered appetite
- Weight loss

- Chronic constipation
- Vomiting
- Fatigue
- Chronic diarrhea
- Irritability
- Malnourishment

In teens, manifestations of celiac disease can also include:

- Depression
- Growth problems
- Delayed puberty
- Dermatitis herpetiformis
- Canker sores

As for adults, common manifestations of celiac disease include:

- Bone loss and osteoporosis
- Joint and bone pain
- Arthritis
- Depression
- Anxiety
- Seizures
- Hands and feet numbness
- Irregular menstruations
- Canker sores
- Dermatitis herpetiformis

How is the celiac disease treated?

As with other autoimmune disorders, there's no permanent cure for celiac disease, this ailment being kept under control by avoiding and completely removing foods that contain gluten from the sufferer's diet. Although recently a group of scientists developed a vaccine that seems to stop the body's reaction to gluten, studies are still needed to prove the effectiveness of this treatment against gluten intolerance.

Until new treatments will be developed, the gluten-free diet remains the only reliable solution to gluten sensitivity. This not only prevents the unpleasant symptoms caused by gluten intake but also helps the villi and microvilli of the cells in the intestinal tract recover, so the digestive system gets healed in time.

However, switching to a gluten-free diet isn't as simple as it sounds and most people give up gluten progressively, which isn't healthy as even the smallest amount of this compound can trigger the typical manifestations. The gluten-free diet will be described later in this report.

In some people, gluten intolerance and celiac disease cause other health issues, so in order to keep symptoms of CD under control, additional treatments may be required. These treatments usually include vaccinations for flu, the HIB/MenC vaccine against pneumonia, sepsis and meningitis and pneumococcal vaccine, protecting against infections triggered by the Streptococcus pneumoniae bacterium.

Nutritional supplements can also help the digestive system repair faster and they prevent nutritional deficiencies caused by CD, such as anemia. In people who develop dermatitis herpetiformis as a consequence of gluten intolerance, prescribed medication may also be needed.

What foods can celiac disease sufferers eat?

Celiac disease sufferers are allowed to eat absolutely all foods that don't contain gluten, from eggs, beans, nuts and seeds in unprocessed form, fish, poultry and other fresh, non-breaded meat, to veggies, fruits and dairy products.

Contrary to the general opinion, grains aren't completely forbidden to CD sufferers. There are actually lots of products in this category that are safe for people with gluten intolerance, and these include:

- non-contaminated corn and cornmeal,
- buckwheat,
- flax,
- arrowroot,

- amaranth,
- millet,
- non-contaminated rice,
- quinoa,
- soy,
- sorghum,
- teff,
- tapioca,
- gluten-free flours

Baking soda, dal, gelatin, kudzu, chick peas, lentils, peanuts, peas, gram, channa, potato starch and flour, spices, tofu, yam, yeast and all products that have not been cross-contaminated can be safely consumed by people suffering from celiac disease. On the other hand, healthy products that have been contaminated can trigger the specific CD symptoms in celiac suffers, therefore should be avoided. Such products include:

- Meat cooked on a grill that hasn't been cleaned after a product containing gluten was grilled.

- Gluten-free products that have been milled using the same equipment that has been used for processing foods containing gluten.

- Products in bulk bins that have been handled with the same scoops used for gluten-rich foods.

- Gluten-free pasta or rice cooked in the same water with products containing gluten.

- Gluten-free foods cooked in oil that has been used for frying products containing gluten.

- Candies or cereals bought in bulk, as bins and scoops may not have been cleaned after non-gluten-free items have been handled.

Besides these foods, people who suffer from gluten sensitivity should also question a series of products that are on the gluten-free list in most cases, but might contain gluten, depending on the producer. Labels should be carefully read when buying:

- Flavored yogurts may contain wheat bran, cookie crumbs or granola, which may contain gluten.

- Sauces for nachos, shredded cheese and cheese spreads may be thickened with wheat flour or starch, which may contain gluten.

- Buckwheat flour and pasta, rice mixes, corn cereals, multigrain cakes, rice crackers and other similar products may contain gluten, depending on the producer.

- Imitation fish products may contain wheat starch.

- Roasted nuts and seeds may contain wheat starch or wheat protein, so labels should be double checked before buying these products.

- Meat substitutes like vegetarian burgers for example may contain non-GF wheat flour or starch.

- Dates may be dusted with non-FG flour.

- Canned or dried soups may contain wheat flour.

- Cake icings and frostings may be made with wheat starch.

- Chips and tacos may be made with wheat flour or starch.

Can a non-celiac develop gluten intolerance?

Gluten intolerance can be present in non-celiac people, the celiac disease being the result and not the cause of gluten intolerance. In other words, people that are sensitive to gluten can be celiacs or non-celiacs, so the answer to this question is yes, a non-celiac can develop gluten intolerance. However, symptoms of gluten sensitivity will be slightly different in people with CD and non-celiac sufferers.

To correctly diagnose their condition, people suspecting they're celiacs or intolerant to gluten should start by removing all sources of gluten from their diet. If they notice improvements in their health state after a week or so, then the intolerance to gluten is confirmed. However, special tests are needed in order to see if the symptoms are caused by gluten intolerance or celiac disease.

Unfortunately, the celiac disease can't be diagnosed based on symptoms only so blood tests and biopsy are needed for detecting this ailment. Unlike gluten intolerance, celiac disease is a more severe condition caused by an immunity problem, so diagnosing this ailment requires a more complex approach.

Is gluten intolerance the same with wheat allergy?

Gluten intolerance is the term used for describing the body's inability to process gluten, so this health issue refers strictly to this specific protein. Wheat allergy on the other hand defines the allergic reaction that can be caused by any ingredient in wheat.

The allergic reaction is the response – a very rapid and serious one – from your immune system, and usually manifests as a rash, itching or wheezing. The intolerance doesn't necessarily manifest through such symptoms; in these cases, manifestations develop more slowly, often many hours after eating the wheat products.

Wheat allergy is one of the most common food allergies in children, avoiding products containing wheat being the solution to keeping symptoms under control. In some cases, medications are also necessary, especially in kids who accidentally eat wheat. Such products include bread, breakfast cereals, crackers and cakes, pasta, soy sauces, condiments, ketchup and beer.

Although wheat allergy is sometimes confused with celiac disease and gluten intolerance, these aren't the same ailment. In people with wheat allergy, the body starts producing antibodies to more types of proteins found in wheat, while in celiac disease, only antibodies to gluten are produced in the small intestine.

A person who's intolerant to gluten may not have any reaction when using a lipstick that contains gluten or another wheat derivative, but people who are allergic to wheat can experience very unpleasant symptoms when using such products.

How is celiac disease diagnosed?

To diagnose the celiac disease specific tests are needed, as unlike gluten intolerance, this ailment is caused by an immunity problem so it's not only the result of an inflamed or too sensitive digestive tract.

People suspected to have celiac disease should initially take some blood tests for specific antibodies. Antibodies are proteins produced inside the human organism, by the immune system, whose role is to fight bacteria, viruses and other pathogens that could cause health issues. In certain conditions, the organism produces antibodies against substances that aren't actually harmful or even against its own cells. This is how autoimmune disorders appear.

People with celiac disease have abnormally elevated levels of tTGA (anti-tissue transglutaminase antibodies) and EMA (anti-endomysium antibodies). If the results of the blood test are negative, the subject might be gluten intolerant without being a celiac.

Another diagnostic test for celiac disease is the intestinal biopsy for which a small biopsy is taken from the walls of the small intestine. This tissue sample is then examined for checking the potential damages of villi and microvilli. If cells in the intestinal tissues are healthy, then patient doesn't have celiac disease.

How is gluten intolerance diagnosed?

Gluten intolerance is different from the celiac disease, as it isn't necessarily caused by or linked with an immunity disorder. People who are intolerant to gluten may or may not be celiacs, so this is why diagnosis is slightly different. Obviously, you can start with a biopsy and blood test to make sure you aren't affected by celiac disease, but usually these aren't the first measures people take when they first notice they experience unpleasant symptoms after eating products that contain gluten.

Most people start by removing gluten-based products from their diet, this being actually the easiest way to diagnose gluten intolerance at home, without special tests. If by removing all the foods containing gluten from their diet, one realizes the symptoms no longer appear, then the gluten intolerance is almost confirmed. At this point, besides sticking with the new regimen, one should also do the previously mentioned tests to see if they're celiacs or not.

CHAPTER 3: The Gluten-Free Diet

What is a gluten-free diet?

A gluten-free diet is, in the simplest terms possible, a diet that excludes foods containing gluten, mostly wheat-based products, barley, rye and triticale-based products. The main goal and indication of a gluten-free diet is the treatment of the celiac disease, ailment characterized by the inflammation of the small intestine due to gluten intake.

By eliminating the main cause of the symptoms specific to celiac disease or gluten intolerance, the gluten-free diet helps people suffering from increased sensitivity to gluten to have an almost-normal life and experience fewer symptoms or complications. However, in some cases the gluten-free diet isn't enough, a more powerful treatment that suppresses the immune system being necessary.

The gluten-free diet is quite restrictive when followed correctly, as it's important for people with gluten intolerance to completely avoid this compound in order to keep symptoms away. Here are the foods that should be completely avoided, as they contain gluten in most cases:

- barley,
- rye,
- wheat,
- triticale.

Still, avoiding wheat can be quite tricky given the wide range of products containing wheat derivatives. Thus, in case you're unsure about a product and not enough information is available on the label, it's better to avoid it if it's included in the following categories:

- graham flour,
- farina,
- bulgur,
- kamut,
- durum flour,
- spelt,
- semolina.

Unless labeled gluten-free (GF), you should also avoid:

- cakes,
- cereals,
- pies,
- candies,
- cookies,
- croutons,
- crackers,
- graham breads,
- French fries,
- pastas,
- matzo,
- imitation meat,
- gravies,
- salad dressings,
- rice mixes,
- soy sauce,
- tortilla chips,
- soup bases,
- vegetables in sauce.

- Oats are often contaminated with gluten so even if they don't contain this compound by themselves, it's better to remove these products from your diet as well.

Is the gluten-free diet for everyone?

Everyone can embrace the gluten-free lifestyle, but this isn't necessary for all people out there unless they actually have gluten sensitivity, are gluten intolerant or have wheat allergy or celiac disease. The gluten-free diet is often seen as a fad, especially because lots of celebrities started promoting this diet as a miraculous weight loss solution.

Yes, gluten-free is better for some people, but can be a struggle for others, as eating only foods free of gluten is surely more costly than having a regular diet. Obviously, the GF diet is the one you should embrace if eating gluten causes bloating, cramps, discomfort, dizziness, vomiting, nausea and any other symptom from the ones mentioned in the previous sections of this report.

Still, if you're only willing to go gluten-free in order to drop excess pounds, you should first ask your doctor if this is really the best solution. Does this mean gluten-free can be unhealthy in some cases? Yes, it can, and here's the explanation!

Given the increasing popularity of gluten-free products, lots of producers are trying to make their GF foods tastier and more attractive, so they add extra sugar or fats to enhance the taste and add more flavor to their products. Obviously, this makes lots of gluten-free foods – which should theoretically be healthier – unhealthier than gluten-rich ones, and instead of losing weight you can actually gain some pounds after going gluten-free.

To conclude: the gluten-free diet isn't for those looking for a weight loss method but for those who actually are sensitive to gluten and need to eat healthier in order to avoid the unpleasant symptoms of gluten intolerance.

Nutritional effects of gluten-free diet

The first and most obvious effect of a gluten-free diet is the removal of most products containing wheat, barley, rye and other similar ingredients from their diet. The intake of grains is drastically reduced so people who go gluten-free often look for alternatives and substitutes. The bad part is nutritional deficiencies can appear by removing all grains from one's diet, as grains and cereals are often the main sources for some minerals and vitamins.

On the other hand, these deficiencies can be prevented by replacing the gluten-based foods with products that provide the same nutrients. For example, if the intake of vitamin B is reduced after removing grains from your diet, you can prevent a deficiency by simply increasing the intake of veggies and fruits containing this vitamin.

Then, gluten is surely not the only culprit behind weight gain, bloating, abdominal discomfort, cramps, gas, constipation and other digestive issues that people deal with these days. This means that simply removing gluten from your diet and going gluten-free won't do such a drastic change in your overall health state if your excess weight or digestive problems or dizziness and increased tiredness are caused by another factor.

A gluten-free diet will ensure a better absorption of nutrients through the mucous membrane of the small intestine as the cells forming this membrane will recover and their normal function will be restored. But if you're also lactose intolerant for example, the nutritional effects of a gluten-free diet will not be as impressive unless you also remove dairy products from your menu.

The gluten-free diet can be beneficial or harmful if you're not approaching the new lifestyle the right way. Many grains are enriched with vitamins as said, so if you're not eating these products anymore you might need to supplement the intake of these nutrients.

Calcium, iron, niacin, folate, thiamin, riboflavin and fibers are only some of the nutrients you might miss if removing grains from your diet, so you might want to just look for some gluten-free versions of these foods instead of completely removing them from your menu. Make sure to always check labels when buying gluten-free foods, as these – as previously said – can be quite rich in sugars and fats.

Benefits of a gluten-free diet

Going gluten-free can significantly change your health. In many individuals the excess pounds start "melting down" once gluten is removed from their menu and a cleaner and healthier diet is adopted. But weight loss is not the only benefit people experience after switching to a GF diet. Here are the most common benefits of this eating strategy:

- Gluten-free diets reduce the likelihood of developing inflammatory conditions therefore lots of ailments can be prevented by simply eliminating this ingredient from your diet.

- Going gluten-free improves digestion and absorption of nutrients, enhancing one's energy levels and reducing the risks of eating emotionally, of developing nutritional deficiencies or eating disorders. Also, it reduces hunger pangs as it helps one cope with their cravings better.

- Gluten-free ensures lower cholesterol and blood sugar levels when done correctly, as it implies a higher intake of fruits and veggies and a lower intake of products that might alter the levels of cholesterol and glucose in blood.

- A diet that's poorer in gluten is usually higher in fibers coming from fruits, veggies and legumes, as well as in proteins, so it's easier to build a leaner and stronger body once gluten is given up.

- Immunity is strengthen by removing gluten, as the body no longer needs to produce antibodies when grains are eaten, so the functioning of immune cells gets healthier.

- Risk of arthritis and other ailments affecting the joints and bones gets lower once the compound triggering inflammatory processes in these areas is removed from one's diet.

- Risk of allergies is reduced by going gluten free as lots of people develop allergies to wheat products in time.

- Skin improves as blood sugar levels are regulated and inflammatory processes are less likely to occur.

- Rosacea and acne outbreaks are less often once going gluten free, as the delivery of nutrients, water and oxygen to skin is enhanced, thus skin cells become healthier.

- Last, gluten-free relieves the symptoms of celiac disease and gluten intolerance, this being probably the most important benefit of removing this ingredient from one's diet.

-

Side effects of a gluten-free diet

We said before that the gluten-free diet can be harmful in some people, the main problem with GF being the potential nutritional deficiencies this diet can cause. People that go gluten-free tend to completely avoid grains, when there are actually lots of products in this category that can be consumed. These products are labeled gluten-free or are naturally free of gluten, so a good strategy for eliminating only those grains that are actually unhealthy for you is to create your personalized list of allowed and not allowed grains.

The basic principles of eating healthy and adopting a balanced diet does not change just because you decide going gluten-free. You can still cause a lot of damage to your body if you keep in your menu products like "gluten-free" cookies, ice-creams, crackers and flours and if your diet consists mostly of highly processed foods, rich in fats and sugars. Healthier should mean less processed and more natural or organic, not gluten-free necessarily.

If you go gluten-free and forget to check your levels of vitamins and minerals you expose yourself to an increased risk of developing various health problems, from the simplest skin problems to more serious ailments. Here are some of the side effects gluten-free diets can cause:

- Unless you pay attention to the fiber intake after going gluten-free, you might experience constipation and digestive issues more often, as for lots of people grains are among the first sources of fibers.

- Another unpleasant effect is that your sensitivity to gluten cross-contamination may significantly increase after going gluten-free, which means your body can react a lot worse when eating even a small piece of a product that has been contaminated with gluten, even if you're not a celiac or allergic to gluten.

- You'll most probably see fluctuations in your weight after switching to a GF diet. For some people, this means losing the excess pounds in time, but for other it just means putting on extra kilos, due to a higher intake of fats and sugars and a lower intake of filling fibers.

- You might discover you're also lactose intolerant so you might need to give up milk and dairy products as well. This isn't necessarily bad, but then you'll have to put a lot more effort in preventing nutritional deficiencies as lots of the nutrients in milk, dairy and grains will have to be supplied through other sources or through dietary supplements.

- Given that you'll most probably get a lower amount of vitamins after going gluten-free, you'll need to watch the intake of these nutrients more carefully, especially for vitamin B.

On the other hand, lots of people decide trying it but don't pay enough attention to the products they eat and end up buying products that aren't actually free of gluten. As a result, they live with the impression that gluten free isn't actually good for them and they continue to blame the poor protein in grains for their abdominal discomfort, pain, dizziness, headaches or weight gain. So these might also be side effects of GF if you're not doing it the right way.

From the financial point of view, gluten-free is more costly so you might also see this as a "side-effect", an undesirable one most probably.

It's therefore recommended to analyze absolutely all these aspects carefully and see if the benefits outweigh the side effects in your case and if it's really worth going gluten-free or if you just need to eat a little cleaner and healthier.

How to correctly start the gluten-free diet?

Like any other important change, switching to a gluten-free diet after years of eating "with gluten" might not be exactly what your body looks for, so you shouldn't be surprised if your body doesn't react very well after the first gluten-free days. It does take time for your body to get used to the new eating habits so you should take it progressively and unless you're allergic to gluten or suffering from celiac disease, you can try to remove gluten-rich products from your menu gradually.

Obviously, it's a lot better to completely give up gluten from the start, but lots of people find this hard and they feel deprived, hungry, moody, irritable and nervous after the first days of gluten-free. But there's a very simple solution to these problems: nowadays there are lots of GF products, even pasta and bread, so you do have a wide range of products to choose from if you're ready to pay the costs. The gluten-free diet is definitely more costly than any regular diet that includes normal bread, so make sure you're well aware of this aspect before going GF.

In case you already analyzed the benefits and unpleasant aspects of switching to a gluten-free diet and you're sure you want to change your eating habits and adopt this strategy, here's what you should do:

- Get diagnosed and find out if you're a celiac, have gluten intolerance or just have other digestion problem that's causing you the unpleasant symptoms that made you decide to switch to a gluten-free lifestyle. You might lose motivation in time if you don't have a really good reason to stick to GF.

- Learn to shop correctly. Read labels and ask for gluten-free products when ordering something at restaurants or bakery departments. Lots of supermarkets have special corners for GF products so make sure to ask for those if you're not able to find the products you need. If you want to save time you can always browse online for shops offering gluten-free products.

- Focus more on real food and unprocessed products as these are more likely to be gluten-free and not contaminated with gluten compared to processed ones. Also, these are usually healthier, richer in nutrients and poorer in calories than processed foods.

- Avoid buying from bulk bins as cross-contamination is a real problem and you might end up buying something that's not actually gluten-free.

- Find healthy replacements, such as gluten-free flours or eggs for thickening your dishes.

- Browse for creative gluten-free recipes and experience more in the kitchen, as otherwise your dishes might suddenly become a lot more boring and you'll surely find it difficult to stick with gluten-free foods if you'll only eat veggies and fruits in their simplest form.

- Prepare your own dishes when traveling and make sure to always check labels if buying products from airports, supermarkets, gas stations and so on, as you still have to stick with your gluten-free regimen even while traveling if you really want to see improvements in your health.

What to incorporate in a gluten-free diet?

The answer to this question depends on the reason you're going gluten-free. If you take this decision due to an increased sensitivity to gluten, to wheat allergy or celiac disease, then it's surely recommended to only incorporate in your diet those foods that are completely anti-inflammatory and auto-immune, meaning that they won't cause any reaction from your immune system and won't affect the cells within your digestive tract and small intestine.

Foods you can safely incorporate in your diet in whatever amount you decide, in this case, include:

- fruits high in fibers,
- vegetables,
- nuts,
- chicken,
- fish and any other lean meat,
- olive or coconut oil.

> Try eating only foods in these categories for a couple of days, just to see if your health issues were really caused only by gluten. If they weren't, you'll most probably continue to experience bloating, cramps, low energy levels and headaches even after removing the so called triggers.

What else can you incorporate in your gluten-free diet? As said, products labeled "gluten-free" can generally be safely consumed but if there's no such label on a product, make sure to check all the other ingredients and to ask your doctor's advice or to do your own research in order to see whether those ingredients might have been contaminated with gluten in the production process.

Oats for example can be good or bad, depending on how they're processed. Cross-contamination appears in lots of cases, when gluten-free foods come into contact with products containing gluten, so unless the oats package is labeled GF, it's better not to buy it. As a general rule, incorporate in your menu only those foods that are naturally free of gluten or that are labeled gluten free, and question absolutely all the other products.

Here's a more detailed list of foods that are naturally free of gluten:

- Eggs
- Beans

- Amaranth
- Buckwheat
- Arrowroot
- Coconut
- Carob
- Cornstarch and corn
- Poultry
- Fish
- Seafood
- Millet
- Milk
- Lentils
- Nuts
- Potatoes
- Herbs
- Spices
- Fresh fruits
- Vegetables
- Fresh pork or beef meat
- Canola oil
- Olive oil
- Quinoa
- Rice
- Teff
- Soy
- Tapioca
- Sorghum

Do gluten-free diets support weight loss?

A gluten-free diet can help one lose weight, but this isn't the main purpose of diets restricting the intake of this protein. Gluten-free regimens are designed for people who suffer from the celiac disease or have intolerance to gluten and experience unpleasant symptoms when eating grains or other products containing gluten.

Unless your weight fluctuations aren't actually caused by gluten intake, giving up grains might not bring the expected results, and we'll explain things a little more so that you understand the link between gluten and weight loss.

Going gluten-free can be a good solution for restoring your body's balance, improving your overall health state and losing weight, as long as you don't replace the otherwise healthy grains with products that are labeled GF but are very rich in sugar or fats. A cookie is still a cookie, whether it's gluten-free or not, just like a slice of bread that contains gluten is a lot healthier than a bowl of GF breakfast cereals that are loaded with sugar or artificial flavors or sweeteners.

If you want to make sure you drop pounds while on a gluten-free diet, make sure to get enough fibers from healthy foods and to switch to a protein-rich diet, as otherwise you might experience cravings and hunger pangs really frequently and you might end up eating more than your body actually needs. Fibers and proteins will keep your stomach full and will prevent sugar cravings, which can be quite difficult to handle in the first weeks of your gluten-free lifestyle.

As previously said, once removing gluten from your diet, the mucous membrane lining the small intestine will start absorbing nutrients in a more effective way and this will affect your blood sugar levels as well. This means that if your new diet will be too rich in sugars, you might actually gain weight instead of losing extra pounds, as the excess glucose will be stored as fat unless the body needs it immediately as a source of energy.

How long after going gluten-free will your health improve?

If we refer to celiac disease sufferers who remove gluten from their diet, then changes will be experienced from the first days, as there won't be any other foods to cause them the unpleasant symptoms. However, as previously said, some people who are gluten intolerant are also sensitive to lactose, so it might be necessary to also eliminate milk and dairy products for a period, until the mucous membrane lining the small intestine recovers.

As for weight loss, skin improvement and other similar effects, these will be felt after a longer period, of 3-4 weeks typically, as it takes time for the body to adapt to the new diet. Surely, bloating, gas, diarrhea, constipation or other similar manifestations will disappear or become less frequent once the gluten intake will be reduced, but weight loss won't happen overnight.

CHAPTER 4: Gluten-Free Foods Explained

What nutrients do gluten-free foods contain?

One of the biggest mistakes lots of people do when deciding to go gluten-free is that they completely remove grains from their diet, when this isn't necessary. We already saw there are lots of products in this category that are naturally free of gluten and could be safely consumed. By removing these products, all the vitamins, minerals and fibers provided by grains will disappear from one's diet, which means an increased risk of developing nutritional deficiencies.

Once going gluten-free, you need to make sure you're getting all the nutrients found in the foods you no longer eat from other sources, preferably unprocessed and as poor in chemicals and preservatives as possible. A GF diet needs to provide proteins, fats and carbohydrates, vitamins, minerals and fibers, just like a regular diet.

Fortunately, there are enough products rich in proteins and fibers that don't contain gluten, so the answer to the question above is gluten-free foods can contain all the existent categories of nutrients. Gluten is a protein just like other proteins, so just because a product doesn't contain gluten, it doesn't mean it completely lacks proteins or nutritional value.

Bread made with gluten-free flour is still bread and provides carbohydrates, fibers and vitamins just like regular, gluten-rich bread. Fruits and vegetables are naturally free of gluten but are rich in fibers, vitamins and minerals; meat provides significant amounts of proteins, dairy products are rich in good fats, nuts and seeds also provide proteins, fibers and beneficial oils, so all the important categories of nutrients can be taken from gluten-free products.

What nutrients are missing from gluten-free foods?

As said above, foods that are free of gluten lack just this one nutrient, not all types of proteins, so just because you're switching to a diet that is free of gluten it doesn't mean you completely give up proteins. Actually there's no need to worry you'll develop nutritional deficiencies once switching to gluten-free, if you keep an eye on the foods you're eating and try to make sure you get enough fibers, proteins and vitamins from GF sources, such as lean meat, fruits, legumes and vegetables.

Are gluten-free foods always labeled?

Lots of gluten-free products are properly labeled, but others don't state "gluten-free" on the labels although all the ingredients are listed. So if you want to make sure there's no amount of this protein in the foods you're buying, you need to learn how to read labels and how to recognize products that contain gluten. Some foods do have mentioned on the labels "whole wheat flour" or wheat, barley, rye, oats. These ingredients might contain gluten, so it's better to avoid them unless the products have a "gluten-free" label.

Modified food starch and flavors such as "natural flavor (contains rye)" can also be sources of gluten, so you should also avoid these if you decide going gluten-free. "Unbleached enriched flour" is most probably a source of gluten, just like any other flour obtained from grains containing this protein. So make sure to stay away from products made with such flours as well, unless you see it's clearly mentioned on their labels that those products contain no gluten.

Jumping to fruits and veggies, these are naturally free of gluten so when buying a pack of frozen veggies there's no need to check whether the label says it's free of gluten or not. Obviously, this changes if we're talking about ice-cream, yogurts or other products that contain fruits along with artificial ingredients, such as flavors or thickeners. These are often gluten-rich, so it's better to avoid them.

Are gluten-free foods free from preservatives and additives?

Gluten-free doesn't necessarily mean free of additives, preservatives and other unnecessary and potentially harmful ingredients. Products that are free of gluten can be healthier if you choose vegetables, fruits, meat and dairy, but can also be even worse than the gluten-containing grains, despite of the GF label.

Your body doesn't care if the crackers you're having before lunch have or don't have gluten; the calories still go inside your body and the chemicals in these products remain harmful, even if the products are free of gluten. As previously said, a gluten-free diet can be very healthy or just as unhealthy as a regular regimen, based on foods containing this protein.

Are gluten-free foods free from lactose?

Gluten is a protein, while lactose is a sugar. Gluten is found mostly in grains, lactose is present mostly in cow milk and dairy products. There's no connection between these two compounds, although people with gluten intolerance might also be intolerant to lactose. As previously said in this report, in people who are sensitive to gluten the lining of the small intestine might be damaged.

In this case, gluten molecules aren't properly processed and unpleasant symptoms appear. But the damaged cells of the mucous membrane covering the walls of the digestive tract might also be unable to process lactose, so side effects can be triggered by the intake of this sugar as well.

However, this doesn't mean all products that are free of gluten will also be free of lactose, simply because not all people who suffer from celiac disease or gluten intolerance need to remove milk and dairy from their diet. There are, obviously, products that are naturally free of both these compounds, such as meat for example or legumes, fruits and vegetables, but then again there are also foods that naturally contain one or the other compound.

Milk contains lactose but is free of gluten, so can be safely consumed by celiacs or people with an increased sensitivity to gluten. On the other hand, grains can contain gluten but be free of lactose, so they can be safely consumed by people who are intolerant to lactose. Still, note that people who go gluten-free often become more sensitive to a lot of foods, and milk or other dairy products containing lactose might be among these foods.

If you're concerned about the possibility of being lactose intolerant and gluten intolerant at the same time, you should first remove gluten from your diet and see if your health improves or not, then do the same with lactose-containing products. A week without gluten and lactose should be enough for you to see whether you're experiencing unpleasant symptoms due to gluten only or whether lactose also plays a role in this.

Are there gluten-free fast foods?

There are some places you can get gluten-free menus even if you're into fast food. Dishes free of gluten can vary from salads and baked potatoes to chili, burgers and applesauce, but it's always good to check how those products were prepared, just to make sure they weren't contaminated with gluten.

At Wendy's for example there are quite complex menus especially made for people who are allergic or sensitive to gluten, eggs, milk, fish and soy. Also, Carl's Jr. offers gluten-free fast foods, and Subway has quite a big selection of gluten-free salads.

On the other hand, KFC's or McDonald's menus aren't for people with gluten intolerance, as even if some of their products should be free of gluten, the biggest problem with these foods is cross-contamination. Both potatoes and meat are cooked in hydrogenated oils and menus often contain foods that are rich in chemicals, flavors and other ingredients that are derived from wheat.

Burger King's menus include, at least theoretically, some gluten-free products, although cross-contamination might be present. As for Taco Bell, there are some products free of gluten in their menus, but it's always better to ask before ordering.

Are there vegan gluten-free foods?

Fruits and vegetables are naturally free of gluten, so these two categories should definitely be on your list of groceries if you're a vegetarian going for gluten-free. On the other hand, you shouldn't remove all grains from your menu, as this will seriously affect the intake of vitamins and fibers. The best approach for a vegetarian who switches to a gluten-free diet is to only remove those products that contain gluten, and not to avoid all grains.

There are also lots of replacements, such as soy products, which can be vegetarian and gluten-free at the same time. Also, meat imitations are both vegan and gluten-free, so can be safely consumed by people looking for vegetarian products that won't affect their health state and won't cause the symptoms specific to gluten intolerance.

What are the best gluten-free foods for babies?

When it comes to gluten-free baby food, best choices are always natural ones, such as mashed avocado or bananas, as these are very nourishing and simple to prepare, requiring no cooking and containing no harmful ingredients. Fresh fruits and vegetables are the best although some do require some cooking before being given to babies. Apples and pears for example should be cooked and pureed first.

Meat, even the leanest one, butter, beans and other similar sources or proteins should be avoided at first as they might cause digestive issues. Even if these are free of gluten, they aren't the best choices when it comes to babies so try to stick with simpler products. Baby rice cereal for example is a good alternative and it's free of gluten, so it can be used as replacement for oats or other grains and regular cereals containing gluten. Still, make sure to always wash the dishes and spoons to avoid cross-contamination.

Always keep in mind that solid food shouldn't be given to babies in their first six months of life, as it may cause unpleasant reactions. As for gluten, it's better to avoid it in the first weeks of solid foods and to progressively introduce products containing this protein in your baby's menu. A baby's immune system is a lot more sensitive than an adult's, so it might easily mistake gluten for a virus or pathogen and celiac disease or gluten intolerance can develop.

This rule applies to commercial products as well. It's better to avoid artificial products and highly processed ones even if they're labeled as gluten-free baby food, as your baby's digestive system is just getting used to solid food and needs nutrients, not chemicals and potentially harmful ingredients. If you do want to purchase commercial products to save time and money, make sure to choose more renowned brands and to always check the labels, as this is the best way to avoid gluten and cross-contamination.

Are wheat products the only foods containing gluten?

Contrary to popular belief, gluten isn't found only in wheat and wheat-based products. There are actually lots of other foods that might contain this protein and should be avoided by people suffering from celiac disease or gluten intolerance. The best known sources of gluten are wheat, rye and barley; bread, bread rolls, pudding, cakes, pretzels, dressings and stuffing made with products derived from these grains, muffins, pastry and pancakes can all contain gluten, unless labeled GF.

The much-blamed protein can also be found in pasta, biscuits and cookies, in foods made with couscous, in pizza dough and crumble toppings. Also, batter, scones, breakfast cereals, bagels, muesli, cheesecakes and crumpets can be sources of gluten.

But the presence of this protein in these foods is not really a surprise, so you should always check the labels to make sure you're getting a gluten-free food if you're purchasing one of the products listed above. Unfortunately, there are also a number of foods that are hidden sources of gluten and these are often neglected by people with gluten sensitivity.

While some persons experience no unpleasant symptoms after eating these products, others might have serious reactions to this protein so pay attention and check the labels even if you're buying products that aren't typically associated with gluten or considered typical sources of this protein. Such foods are:

- sausages,
- blue cheese,

- baked beans,
- seitan,
- matzo flour,
- luncheon meat,
- meat pastes,
- pate,
- mustards,
- sauces and soups,
- instant coffee,
- wafers,
- self-basting turkeys,
- brown rice syrup,
- hot chocolate,
- potato chips
- crisps,
- soy sauce,
- licorice,
- salad dressings
- curry powder,
- white pepper,
- malt vinegar
- chutneys can contain gluten or be contaminated with this ingredient.

Can someone on a gluten-free diet eat potatoes?

In their natural form, potatoes are gluten-free so they can be safely consumed by people who are intolerant to gluten or suffer from celiac disease. However, lots or processed products that incorporate potatoes also contain ingredients derived from gluten-based foods. Cross-contamination can also be a problem with potato-based foods, so unless you prepare these foods at home, you should always ask to verify if a dish or product is gluten-free.

Potatoes can successfully replace grains, as they can be used for preparing fulfilling fishes and are a good source of carbohydrates. They can be boiled, steamed, cooked, baked, fried, prepared in the microwave and grilled, so they're very versatile and also easy to prepare.

Very nourishing and rich fibers, potatoes do supply fibers just like grains, but the highest amount of fibers in found in the skin of these veggies. The bad part is some people experience digestive discomfort if potatoes are cooked in their skin, so if you're rather sensitive you should protect your digestive tract by removing skin before preparing potatoes-based dishes.

List of gluten-free foods and ingredients

We previously said that fruits, veggies, fresh meat and milk are naturally free of gluten and can be safely consumed by people with celiac disease or by those with gluten intolerance. However, it's worth giving a more detailed list of foods for each of these categories, just so you see that there are actually lots of alternatives when it comes to eating without gluten.

Gluten-free fruits

All the fruits listed below are naturally free of gluten and should be perfectly safe when washed properly and eaten in their raw state. Canned products, yogurts, puddings and other deserts containing fruits aren't always safe when bought from supermarkets as they might contain thickeners or artificial colors and flavors obtained from wheat and thus containing gluten.
Here are the fruits you can safely eat when raw or incorporated in home-made dishes:

- Apples
- Pears
- Cranberries
- Avocados
- Prunes
- Raspberries
- Blueberries
- Figs

- Plums
- Grapefruits
- Grapes
- Limes
- Pomegranate
- Guava
- Mangos
- Tangerines
- Cantaloupes
- Bananas
- Blackberries
- Nectarines
- Melons
- Oranges
- Rhubarb
- Apricots
- Pineapple
- Peaches
- Papayas
- Lemons
- Quince
- Watermelon

Gluten-free vegetables

Veggies are naturally free of gluten so as long as you cook them at home you can safely eat any product in the list below:

- Asparagus
- Broccoli
- Green beans
- Artichoke
- Cabbage
- Carrots
- Beets
- Brussels sprouts

- Eggplant
- Garlic
- Fennel
- Leafy greens
- Bok choy
- Celery
- Green beans
- Peas
- Cucumbers
- Onions
- Squash
- Parsnips
- Tomatoes
- Potatoes
- Radishes
- Okra
- Rutabaga
- Watercress
- Turnips
- Zucchini

Gluten-free grains and pasta

In what concerns grains, there are lots of products that don't contain gluten in their natural form, so unless you buy them already cooked, the risk of cross-contamination is significantly reduced and these products can be safely consumed:

- Teff
- Millet
- Buckwheat
- Rice
- Soy flour
- Potato starch
- Arrowroot
- Amaranth
- Rice flour
- Corn

- Sago
- Corn flour
- Tapioca
- Gluten-free bread
- GF rolls, crackers, cakes, biscuits and pizza bases
- Rice pasta
- Corn pasta
- Noodles
- Gluten-free pasta
-

Gluten-free meat

Meat is generally gluten-free, except from sausages, pates and burgers which might contain gluten or be contaminated with this ingredient. Then, meat cooked in batter or bread crumbs as well as rissoles, breaded ham and haggis are a source of gluten and should be avoided by people with gluten intolerance. Safe products in this category are fresh meat and poultry, smoked meat, plain cooked meat, all types of fish as long as they're fresh and cooked with GF ingredients, dried fish, smoked fish and fish canned in oil or brine.

Gluten-free dairy products and fats

Products made of milk are generally gluten free, except for the already mentioned yogurts or desserts containing artificial ingredients derived from wheat. Yogurts with cereals or muesli and fromage frais also contain gluten, therefore they should be avoided. As for oats, milk, fruit yogurts, soy and milk desserts and coffee or tea whiteners, these might or might not contain gluten, so labels should be checked before buying these products.

In what concerns the safe, GF dairy products you can incorporate in your menu without worrying about gluten sensitivity, the list includes liquid and dried milk, cheese, cream, sour cream, plain yogurt, buttermilk and plain fromage frais. Butter, margarine, cooking oil and lard are free of gluten as well.

While some beverages, such as beer and malted milk drinks contain gluten and should be removed from your menu if you're intolerant to this protein, others are perfectly safe and can be consumed without any risk. Tea, coffee, fruit juices, cider, sherry, cocoa and GF beer can be part of your menu even if you're a celiac.

As for snacks, homemade rice cakes and crackers, gluten-free crackers and pretzels, seeds, nuts and homemade popcorn are good, gluten-free choices. On the other hand, snacks made of or containing derivatives of wheat, barley and rye should be avoided.

Are gluten-free foods lower in carbs than gluten-based products?

Gluten is a protein so the presence or absence of this ingredient from a product doesn't influence the amount of carbohydrates found in that particular food. It is, however, true that lots of gluten-free foods are poorer in calories, carbohydrates and sugars than foods containing this protein.

Let's take fruits and veggies for example, which are naturally free of gluten and contain lower amounts of carbohydrates than baked deserts or grain-based foods. But if we refer to gluten-based or gluten-free flours, crackers, biscuits, pancakes and other similar products, then the amount of carbohydrates doesn't depend on the presence or absence of gluten.

Are gluten-free foods lower in sugar than gluten-based products?

As previously said, gluten-free foods can be healthier than those products containing this protein, but once again, the amount of sugar found in a dish – whether it's commercial or homemade – doesn't depend on the presence or absence of gluten.

If we refer to baked goods, to pastries, bread, cookies, cakes and other similar products, these can be equally rich in sugar or glucose whether they're gluten-free or gluten-based. On the other hand, if we take vegetables for example, the amount of sugar or glucose is lower than the quantity of sugar found in bread, doughnuts, candies and so on.

What are some good GF replacements for wheat-based thickeners and flours?

The gluten-free diet lacks wheat, rye and barley and all the derivatives, thickeners and flours obtained from these grains. However, it doesn't mean one can no longer eat baked dishes or prepare dressings or sauces that require thickening agents. There are actually lots of gluten-free products that can be successfully used for replacing products that contain gluten.

Given below is a list of good replacements for gluten-based flours and thickeners:

- Arrowroot – this is excellent as thickening substitute and has a neutral flavor compared to gluten-based thickeners. It's also a great choice for people who are trying to avoid potato-based and corn-based foods. This product can be used for desserts as well.

- Tapioca starch is another good alternative to gluten-based starch and can be used for pie fillings, sauces and creamy textures.

- Lotus root flour – although more expensive than other replacements, this thickening agent is easy to digest, nicely colored and excellent for main dishes and desserts. It's free of gluten and can be used to make batter for meat and veggies, to prepare creams and fillings.

- Sorghum flour can successfully replace gluten-based flours and can be used for preparing GF bread or other baked foods. Also, it works great when mixed with other gluten-free flours for adding flavor and texture to dishes.

- Quinoa flour is often used for gluten-free cakes, breads, pancakes or cookies.

- Montina flour is less popular than the previously mentioned products but it's also a very good choice for baked goods. It's obtained from a plant originating in North America and it's quite similar to millet.

Is malt vinegar free of gluten?

- Depending on the source it's obtained from, malt vinegar can be gluten free. In most cases, this product is obtained from barley so if you're buying pickles, condiments or chutneys, make sure to check the label and in case these products contain malt vinegar, check its source. If it's obtained from barley, don't buy it, it's not gluten-free.

- On the other hand, red wine vinegar, white wine vinegar, cider, sherry and balsamic vinegar are not obtained from barley therefore they are suitable for a gluten-free diet.

Is mustard free of gluten?

Mustard is a plant so the product obtained from the seeds of this plant is naturally free of gluten. However, lots of producers incorporate additional ingredients in their products to change the thickness, flavor and texture of mustards, so it's better to always check the labels and see whether any wheat derivatives are incorporated in the product you want to buy. Wheat flour is quite often used as thickening agent for mustards.

Is glucose syrup free of gluten? What about maltodextrin and dextrose?

Glucose syrup is found in numerous products, mostly sweets, cookies, cakes and candies, but even if it's not the healthiest ingredient, this product is free of gluten so it's safe for celiacs and gluten intolerant people.

Despite its name, maltodextrin is also gluten-free. This product can be obtained from different cereals, from wheat and rice to tapioca and corn, so you can easily find GF versions for this ingredient. Also, dextrose is gluten free, as even if it's obtained from wheat, the production process ensures a final product that contains no gluten.

Is baking powder free of gluten?

Baking powder is obtained from baking soda and cream of tartar, plus an ingredient meant to absorb moisture, that's usually cornstarch. Wheat starch and potato starch can also be used for retaining moisture, so not all brands of baking powder are gluten free. It's therefore necessary to always check the label even when buying a product made by a brand that's generally known to promote gluten-free products.

Can I consume protein powders if I have gluten intolerance?

Protein powders are usually made of whey, which is a protein extracted from milk. Whey provides high-quality amino-acids which are very easy to metabolize and to absorb, so this is why lots or powders for gym goers as well as protein bars and other similar supplements contain whey protein. However, just like the other protein found in milk, casein, whey can cause allergic reactions and is one of the triggers of the unpleasant symptoms experienced by lactose intolerance individuals.

Gluten, although it's not used in protein powders usually, can be present in contaminated whey powder, especially if the same machines are used for packing whey protein and wheat flour during industrial processing of these products. Except for these cases of cross-contamination, whey protein – and implicitly protein powders containing whey – is safe for gluten intolerant people and celiac sufferers.

Still, keep in mind that in celiac disease sufferers, the mucous membrane lining the small intestine is damaged and this can result in lactose intolerance as well. This means that even if celiacs aren't necessarily intolerant to lactose and whey, they can experience side effects when using protein powders if their digestive tract develops an increased sensitivity to this ingredient or is too damaged due to the celiac disease.

CHAPTER 5: Gluten-Free Recipes

Cooking at home and preparing your own snacks, desserts and lunch meals for office is the best way of avoiding gluten whether you're a celiac disease sufferer or you're just trying to remove this ingredient from your menu in order to get rid of the unpleasant digestive symptoms gluten intolerance can trigger.

Until now we said most fruits, veggies, meat and dairy products are free of gluten, but eating only raw fruits and legumes or freshly cooked meat doesn't really sound like a long-term solution, so taking a look at the following gluten-free recipes can be extremely helpful especially if you're looking for variety in your diet. Gluten-free doesn't have to mean tasteless or boring, as even if you'll be avoiding most grains, cereals and pastries, you can still prepare lots of tasty, nourishing and fulfilling foods.

Every day gluten-free recipes for breakfast

For lots of people breakfast is the meal that's the richest in gluten, as the highest quantity of bread is consumed at the first meal of the day. However, going gluten-free doesn't have to mean skipping breakfast. There are actually lots of alternatives when it comes to having a healthy, gluten-free breakfast, so before describing some recipes, we'll just list some solutions for a GF breakfast.

First, you can prepare a fruit-based breakfast, like a fresh fruit salad, a fresh smoothie, homemade applesauce or banana and avocado puree. Then, you can have a gluten-free omelet with smoked fish and veggies or, if you're willing to spend more money on food, some gluten-free bread with homemade peanut butter or cheese cream and tomatoes.

Gluten-free pancakes (serves 8)

Pancakes are a great alternative for breakfast and can be safely consumed by people who are intolerant to gluten, as long as the recipe uses specific, GF ingredients. Here's a quick recipe for gluten-free blueberry pancakes.

Ingredients needed:

- 1 ½ cup of fresh or frozen blueberries,
- 2 eggs,
- 2 ½ cups gluten-free flour, such as sorghum flour or buckwheat flour
- 1 cup of buttermilk,
- 4 tbsp. of softened butter,
- 2 tbsp. of olive oil,
- 3 tsp. GF baking soda,
- 2 tbsp. sugar,
- 1 tsp. vanilla extract.

Method: In a medium sized bowl, mix the softened butter with eggs and sugar. In a larger bowl, mix the GF flour and the baking soda, then add the vanilla extract and buttermilk and continue mixing until all ingredients are blended. Add all the ingredients in the larger bowl and blend again until you obtain a thick paste. You can change the texture and thickness of your pancakes by adding some milk or water.

On medium heat, melt the remaining butter in a pancake skillet and spoon 1/3 cup of the pancake batter. Smooth the pancake and dot the top with blueberries, then cook until slightly golden. Flip the pancake and cook on the other side until golden. Serve warm or cold!

Important tip: make sure that all the utensils and pans you're using are perfectly clean and free of gluten. Read labels for all the products you're using and in case you're not sure a product is gluten-free, replace is with one that has a GF label.

Vegetable breakfast mix (serves 4)

For those who want a lighter breakfast, a mix of veggies, freshly baked, can also be a great choice. Here's a quick recipes for 4 people.

Ingredients needed:

- 4 eggs,
- 4 large Shiitake mushrooms, thinly sliced
- 200 grams of spinach,

- 8 tomatoes, thinly sliced
- 1 garlic clove, chopped
- 2 tsp. olive oil.

Method: Heat the oven at 180°C. In an ovenproof dish, put the sliced tomatoes and the mushrooms. Cut the garlic into small pieces and place it on top, then drizzle over the oil and add seasonings to taste. Bake for 10 minutes and take out from the oven to add the spinach.

Meanwhile, in a large colander, put the spinach and pour boiling water over it to wilt it. Remove the excess water and add the spinach to the other ingredients, stirring to combine well. Make some small gaps between the veggies and crack the eggs, then return the dish to the oven and cook for another 10 minutes or until the eggs are cooked to your taste. Serve warm!

Tropical smoothie (serves 2)

Ingredients needed:

- 1 large banana, peeled and chopped
- 2 passion fruits, inner fruit only
- 300 ml fresh orange or apple juice,
- 1 small mango or pear, peeled, seeded and diced
- ice cubes.

Method: To prepare this smoothie you'll need a blender. Start by scooping the passion fruits in the blender, and then add the banana, orange juice and mango. Puree the fruits until they're smooth, add the ice cubes and serve. You can also refrigerate the smoothie for later.

Spanish style omelet (serves 8)

Ingredients needed:

- 8 eggs,
- 500 grams potatoes, peeled and cut into 1/8-inch slices
- 2 small onions, peeled and thinly sliced

- knob of butter,
- 1 red pepper, seeded and thinly sliced
- 25 grams chives.

Method: Slice the potatoes, onions and red pepper. Heat the butter in a frying pan at low heat and cook gently until it turns slightly brown. Add the peppers and onions and cook for 5 minutes. In a small bowl, beat the eggs with a fork, add pepper and salt to taste and snip the chives. Stir until well mixed.

In a separate steamer, put the potatoes over the boiling water for 10-15 minutes, until soft. You can also use a regular saucepan if you don't have a steamer; in this case, cover the potatoes with boiling water and simmer for 10 minutes or until cooked. Drain the water.

Heat the oven to medium, add some more butter into the frying pan, put the potatoes, add the onions and peppers on top and pour over the eggs. Place the pan on the top shelf of the oven and cook for 15 minutes or until the omelet gets golden brown. Move the frying pan on a lower rack, cook for 1-2 extra minutes and serve warm.

Quinoa porridge with blueberries (serves 2)

Ingredients needed:

- 1 cup of almond milk,
- ½ cup of water,
- 1 cup fresh blueberries,
- ½ cup GF quinoa,
- ½ tsp. cinnamon,
- 8 almonds,
- 2 tbsp. pumpkin seeds.

Method: In a medium saucepan, mix the almond milk, water and quinoa. Bring to a boil, then reduce to medium-low heat and cover, simmering for 15 minutes or until most of the liquid is absorbed.

Turn off the heat, let it stand for 5 minutes, then stir in the fresh blueberries and add the cinnamon. Stir until well mixed, divide among 2 bowls, top with almonds and pumpkin seeds and serve!

Gluten-free rice pudding (serves 6)

This homemade recipe is very tasty and ideal for breakfast, but make sure to pick gluten-free ingredients!

Ingredients needed:

- 300 grams GF rice,
- 4 cups almond milk,
- 30 g each currants, raisins and almonds,
- 6 whole green cardamom pods,
- 1 tsp. vanilla extract,
- 2 tbsp. maple syrup optionally.

Method: In a pan, add water and bring to boil. Add the almonds and let sit for 1 minute, then drain and slip off the skins. Blend the almonds with the milk until smooth. In a medium saucepan, mix all the ingredients, bring to a boil and reduce the heat to simmer. Stir continuously, mashing any lumps out with a spatula or wooden spoon.

Cover and cook the rice pudding for 20 minutes, stirring occasionally until you obtain the desired thickness. Don't overcook the pudding as it will thicken more once it cools down. Remove from heat, let it cool a little and serve warm. You can add cinnamon powder for extra flavor.

Every day gluten-free recipes for lunch

Chicken with tomatoes and herbs (serves 4)

Ingredients needed:

- 1/4 cup fat free chicken broth,
- 1 small onion, chopped,
- 2 garlic cloves, minced,

- 230 g homemade tomato sauce,
- 1/4 cup red wine vinegar,
- 1/2 tsp. dried oregano,
- 1/2 tsp. dried basil,
- 1/4 tsp. white pepper,
- 4 boneless chicken breasts, skinless.

Method: In large non-stick skillet, heat broth over medium heat. In a different pan or skillet, sauté the onion and garlic for 2 minutes or until tender, then add the tomato sauce, vinegar, oregano, basil and pepper to the onion mix. Add the chicken broth and bring the mixture to boil, and then reduce the heat, stirring occasionally.

Cut the chicken breasts into smaller pieces and add them to the prepared sauce, simmering for 15 minutes and stirring occasionally. Turn the chicken breasts and simmer an additional 30 minutes or until the meat is tender. Serve hot.

Spinach and egg quiche (serves 4)

Ingredients needed:

- ½ red onion, chopped,
- 8 oz. spinach,
- 6 egg whites,
- 2 cloves of garlic chopped fine (sauté in skillet),
- 1/4 cup feta cheese or 1/2 cup ricotta (optional).

Method: Sautee the spinach, garlic, and onion in skillet until spinach wilted. Whisk together the eggs and mix all the ingredients together with the cheese mixture. Add salt and pepper to taste and bake at 170°C for 30 minutes. Serve hot.

Vegetarian beans mixture (serves 4)

Ingredients needed:

- 200 g beans, rinsed and drained,

- 300 g fresh tomatoes, diced,
- 80 g onions, chopped,
- 150 ml water,
- 80 g GF rice,
- 1 tbsp. mustard,
- ¼ tsp. cayenne pepper,
- salt to taste.

Method: In a saucepan with cover, bring water to a boil. Add the rice and return to boil. Reduce heat to low, cover and cook 45 minutes or until rice is cooked and liquid is absorbed. Pour cooked rice into a large bowl and combine with remaining ingredients. Pour into 2-quart baking dish. Bake at 170°C for 2-1/2 hours, stirring occasionally. Serve warm.

Tuna steak with oranges (serves 4)

Ingredients:

- 450 g tuna steaks,
- 60 ml orange juice,
- 1 clove garlic, minced,
- 30 ml olive oil,
- 8 g chopped fresh parsley,
- 15 ml lemon juice,
- 1 g ground black pepper,
- 1 g chopped fresh oregano.

Method: In a large dish, put the orange juice, lemon juice, olive oil, garlic, parsley, oregano and pepper and mix until they combine well. Put the fish steaks in this marinade and turn to coat. Refrigerate the steaks for at least 30 minutes, covering them before placing in the refrigerator.

Meanwhile, preheat the grill at high temperature and oil the grate. Cook each tuna steak for 5 to 6, turning and basting with the marinade on each side. If needed, continue cooking for 5 extra minutes, until you obtain the desired doneness. Remove from the grill, discard the remaining marinade and serve warm.

Chick peas curry (serves 4)

Ingredients:

- 2 tsp. coconut oil,
- 350 g cabbage,
- 180 g onion, diced,
- 180 g sweet bell pepper,
- 180 ml coconut milk,
- 1-2 tsp. garlic, minced,
- 2 tsp. curry powder,
- 400 g chick peas,
- pinch of dried basil,
- salt and pepper to taste.

Method: In a large pan, add oil and sauté the cabbage on medium heat, until it shrinks down. Add the onions and peppers and sauté 3-4 minutes or until just softening. Add the remaining ingredients and stir well.

Cover the pan with a lid and simmer for about 5 minutes until the chick peas are warm. Serve as it is or with baked chicken.

Salmon with asparagus (serves 2)

Ingredients:

- 100 g salmon fillets,
- 2 tsp. ground cumin,
- 2 cups GF rice,
- 2 tbsp. chopped fresh herbs,
- 10 large asparagus stalks,
- 2 tomatoes, diced,
- 2 tbsp. butter

- 20 olives,
- salt and pepper to taste.

Method: Preheat oven to 200⁰C. Using cooking spray, coat a large baking sheet, and then start preparing the salmon fillets by adding salt and pepper on both sides. Rub the mixed herbs into the flesh-side of the salmon fillets and place the fish skin-side down on the baking sheet you prepared and then roast for about 10 minutes or until the fillets are fork-tender.

In the meantime combine the gluten-free rice with the water in a bowl, covering with a lid and microwave on high for 5 minutes then let stand for another 5 minutes. Add herbs, fluff with a fork and season with salt and black pepper. Keep the asparagus in a glass dish with a lid. Dot with pieces of butter then cover and microwave on high for 3 minutes or until the asparagus becomes crisp-tender.

Add the tomatoes and olives in a large bowl. Toss to combine, then season with salt and pepper. Serve the salmon with the rice mixture and asparagus, topped with the tomatoes mixture.

Every day gluten-free recipes for dinner

Sautéed kale (serves 4)

Ingredients:

- 450 g kale, cut into 1 inch strips,
- 2 carrots, sliced,
- 1 small onion, chopped,
- 1 tsp. crushed red pepper flakes,
- 1 garlic clove, diced,
- 1 tbsp. toasted sesame seeds,
- 1/4 cup sliced almonds,

Method: In a large pan, heat the olive oil then add the onion, garlic and red pepper flakes, stirring for about 2 minutes. Add half of the kale, continue stirring for about 1-2 minutes, and then add the rest of the kale. After 6-10 minutes, add the shredded carrots and continue cooking for an additional 2-4 minutes or until kale is tender. Toss in sesame seeds and almonds. Serve!

Lebanese chicken with zucchini and eggplant (serves 4)

Ingredients:

- 400 g skinless chicken breast,
- ½ cup lemon juice,
- 4 cloves garlic, minced
- salt,
- ½ cup olive oil,
- pepper to taste.

  For the veggies:

- 1 cup carrots, peeled and thinly sliced
- 2 cups tomato sauce,
- 1 cup zucchini, thinly sliced
- 1 large eggplant, unpeeled
- 2 cloves garlic, minced
- 1 tbsp. olive oil.

Method: Mix the sea salt and garlic to create a paste for coating the chicken. Add the lemon juice, the olive oil and pepper, mix and coat the skinless chicken breast with this mixture. Refrigerate for 4 to 5 hours so that the meat marinates, then grill the chicken on both sides until golden.

Meanwhile, prepare the veggie mixture. Heat the olive oil and put carrots and zucchini for 3 minutes, cooking at medium heat. Add a few drops of water when the temperature increases. Add tomato sauce and garlic and simmer for 5 minutes.

Grill the unpeeled eggplant on low fire, turning every minute for 5 minutes. Cut the eggplant in half and remove the skin the cut into small cubes. Mix the eggplant with the other ingredients and simmer for another 2 minutes. Serve with the grilled chicken.

Exotic salmon with pineapple (serves 2)

Ingredients:

- 2 salmon fillets, each 120 g,
- 110 ml fresh pineapple juice,
- 225 g diced fresh fruit, such as mango, pineapple or papaya,
- 2 garlic cloves, minced,
- 1/4 tsp. sesame oil,
- 1/4 tsp. ground ginger,
- 2 tbsp. GF soy sauce,
- pepper to taste.

Method: In a small bowl, mix the pineapple juice with soy sauce, garlic and ginger, stirring thoroughly until the ingredients are evenly mixed. Place the salmon fillets in a small baking dish and start pouring the mixture obtained from the pineapple juice over the top of the fillets. Put the fish in the refrigerator and let it marinate for about 1 hour. Turn the salmon fillets periodically.

Meanwhile, preheat the oven to 170°C. Using cooking spray, coat two squares of aluminum foil and place the salmon fillets on these foils. Drizzle each fish fillet with 1/8 teaspoon sesame oil, then sprinkle with salt and pepper and add ½ cup of diced fruits on the top of each salmon fillet.

Wrap the aluminum foil around the salmon fillets, folding the edges down to seal so that the fillets will cook evenly. Put in the oven and bake for about 10 minutes on each side or until the salmon is opaque when tested with a fork. Place the salmon fillets to individual plates and serve immediately.

Gluten-free turkey pizza

Ingredients:

- 1 pre-baked gluten-free pizza crust,
- 6 slices turkey,
- 12 tsp. olive oil,
- 4 cloves of garlic, minced,
- 1 tsp. fresh oregano, chopped.

Method: Preheat oven to 200°C and in case you have a special pizza stone, make sure to place it in oven to preheat. You can also use a regular baking sheet or a round pan if you don't have a pizza stone. To prepare the dish, brush each crust with olive oil and sprinkle minced garlic all over the crust. Place the turkey slices evenly and sprinkle herbs on pizza crust.

Bake in preheated oven for about 10-12 minutes and crust is golden brown.

Chicken salad (serves 2)

Ingredients needed:

- 1 bell pepper, any color,
- 180 g skinless chicken breast,
- 1/2 large sweet onion,
- 2 cups lettuce,
- 2 tbsp. olive oil.

Method: Slice the bell pepper and onion into thin strips and place them in a skillet, tossing with olive oil. Turn on medium heat and add salt, cooking until the veggies get soft. This shouldn't take more than 20 minutes. Meanwhile, until the vegetables are well cooked, start preparing the chicken breasts – cook it in the oven or on the grill preferably. Rub salt and pepper onto the breast before placing on the grill or in a skillet and cook until fully white inside. When the meat is ready, slice it into strips.

Prepare two salad bowls with 1 cup lettuce each. Divide the veggies and chicken into the two bowls and toss- and eat! You can add homemade tomato sauce and GF rice.

Spicy potatoes (serves 2)

Ingredients:

- 225 g potatoes, cut into small pieces,
- 1 1/2 tsp. paprika,
- 1 tsp. salt,
- 1 1/2 tsp. ground cumin,
- 1 tsp. ground fennel,
- 1/2 tsp. ground ginger,
- 1 tsp. chili powder,
- 2 tbsp. olive oil.

Method: In a bowl, combine the potatoes and 1/2 tbsp. oil. In another bowl, mix the ground cumin, ginger, fennel, paprika, chili powder and salt. Put this mixture over the potatoes and toss well until they're fully coated. Place the potatoes on an aluminum foil and seal the packet.

Grill the potatoes in foil for about 15-20 minutes, until they are well-cooked and look tender. Drizzle the potatoes with the remaining olive oil and then transfer them to a serving bowl. Serve warm, with chicken or salmon.

Gluten-free soup recipes

Tomato soup

Ingredients:

- 400 g tomatoes,
- 2 tsp. butter,
- sea salt and pepper to taste,
- mint leaves,
- coriander leaves.

Method: Put the tomatoes in boiling water (3 cups) for 2 minutes. Transfer them to ice-cold water immediately. Peel the skins and cut the tomatoes into small pieces. Take water in a pan, let it boil. Add the chopped tomatoes. Add mint and salt to the boiling mixture.

Boil for about 5-6 minutes. Allow it to cool and blend the tomatoes with the help of a mixer. Sieve the blended mixture to remove the seeds. Garnish it with a dash of butter and coriander leaves. Serve hot.

Squash soup

Ingredients:

- 2 tbsp. extra-virgin olive oil,
- 1 onion, diced,
- 1 tsp. shredded ginger root,
- 4 cups oven cooked butternut squash,
- 4 cups chicken broth, low in sodium,
- salt and pepper to taste.

Method: To cook the squash, cut it length wise, take out the seeds and place in the oven on a cookie sheet, bake for approx. 1 hour at 170°C. Heat the oil in a large soup pot. Add onion and ginger and cook until softened. Add squash, onions, ginger, chicken broth and pulse/puree in blender. Add to large pot to reheat and salt and pepper to taste.

Chickpeas soup

Ingredients:

- 200 g chickpeas, rinsed and drained,
- 400 g tomatoes, whole or chopped,
- 140 g red split lentils,
- 2 tsp. cumin seeds,
- 850 ml vegetable stock,
- small bunch coriander,
- large pinch chili flakes,

- 1 tbsp. olive oil,
- 1 red onion, thinly sliced
- 4 tbsp. Greek yogurt.

Method: Place a large saucepan on medium heat and dry-fry the chili flakes and cumin seeds for about 1 minute or until they start releasing their aromas. In the same pan, add the olive oil and onions and cook for about 5 minutes. When onion is soft, stir in the lentils, tomatoes and stock veggies and bring to the boil. Simmer for about 15 minutes or until the lentils are soft.

Mix the soup using a stick blender or place it in a food processor and mix until it becomes a rough purée. Transfer the soup back into the pan, then stir in chickpeas. Heat the dish, season to taste and stir in the coriander. To serve, add a dollop of yogurt and top with coriander leaves. Serves 5-6 persons.

Gluten-free dessert recipes

Fruit salad (8 cups)

Ingredients:

- 1 peeled, cored pineapple,
- 3 mangos (3 cups/675 gm.), chopped
- 2 papaya (2 cups/450gm),
- 3 ripe kiwi,
- 2 cups/450gm chopped strawberries,
- 2 bananas, sliced thin,
- 1 juiced orange (about 1/3 cup/70 gm.),
- unsweetened shredded coconut (optional).

Method: Squeeze orange and make a sauce in blender by mixing orange juice with 1 cup chopped strawberries and 1 cup chopped mango. Peel, chop and mix rest of fruit in large bowl. Pour sauce over fruit and mix. Sprinkle coconut over each serving.

Grilled pineapple

Ingredients for the marinade:

- 1 tbsp. olive oil,
- 1 firm pineapple,
- 1/4 tsp. ground cloves,
- 1 tbsp. fresh lime juice,
- 1 tbsp. grated lime zest,
- 1 tsp. ground cinnamon,

Method: Heat the grill. In a bowl, combine the lime juice, olive oil, cinnamon and cloves, and whisk to blend. Set aside to make the marinade.

Start preparing the pineapple by cutting off the base of the fruit and the crown of the leaves. Stand the pineapple upright and pare off the skin using a sharp and large knife. To make this easier, cut downward in long, vertical strips, just below the fruit's surface. Stand the fruit upright after removing the peel and cut it lengthwise, in half.

Continue cutting the fruit, this time placing each pineapple half cut-side down and slicing it lengthwise into 4 pieces. Place the fruit pieces in the bowl with the marinade and start stirring to coat the fruit well. When fully coated, transfer the pineapple on the grill and cook for about 5 minutes, basting 1-2 times more with the remaining marinade.

Cook thoroughly then transfer the pineapple to a different part of the grill, where temperature is slightly lower. Continue grilling the pineapple, basting again with marinade. When the pineapple is golden and tender, remove it from the grill and place it on plates. Sprinkle with the lime zest and serve warm.

Gluten-free muffins (makes 10-12 muffins)

Ingredients:

- 2 cups GF oats blended into a powder,

- 1 tsp. baking powder,
- ¼ cup unsweetened applesauce,
- 1 cup milk,
- 1/3 cup cottage cheese,
- 1 egg,
- 1 tbsp. vanilla extract,
- ½ cup GF flour, such as buckwheat flour
- ½ tsp. salt

Method: Pre-heat the oven to 350-degrees F (170-degrees C) and pour all the ingredients into a blender, mixing at high speed until they form a smooth paste. You can mix in fruits by hand or include them in the blender; blueberries work best but you can also incorporate apples, strawberries, raspberries or pears. Pour the obtained paste into a muffin tin greased with coconut oil. Cook the muffins until the toothpick comes out clean, for about 40 minutes. Serve cold or warm.

Apple cobbler (makes 6 servings)

Ingredients:

- 1 lb. peeled and chopped apples,
- 1 cup pear or berries or whatever fruit you prefer,
- ½ cup gluten-free oatmeal,
- 1 tbsp. cinnamon,
- ¼ cup gluten-free flour, such as almond flour
- ¼ cup chopped dates,
- 1/8 cup chopped almonds.

Method: Preheat the oven to 350 degrees. In a bowl, mix together the peeled and chopped apples, the berries and dates and stir until well combined. Pour the mixture into a baking dish and sprinkle with cinnamon. Mix the flour, oatmeal and almonds in a separate bowl until well combined and sprinkle on top of the fruits and bake for about 25-30 minutes or until lightly browned. You can top with Greek yogurt & honey.

Pumpkin cheesecake

Ingredients for crust:

- 1½ cup finely chopped walnuts,
- 2 tbsp. coconut oil,
- 2 tbsp. honey.

Method: Press all the above ingredients together and press in the bottom of your pie pan. It will seem not fully compact, but once you add pie filling, it all comes out nicely after cooking.

Ingredients for filling:

- 8 oz. low fat cream cheese,
- 8 oz. plain Greek yogurt,
- ½ cup 100% pure maple syrup,
- 1/3 cup pureed pumpkin,
- ½ tsp. vanilla,
- ¼ tsp. cinnamon and nutmeg.

Method: Blend until smooth, pour into piecrust and bake for 50 minutes at 350-degrees F.

CHAPTER 6: Potential Obstacles in Going Gluten-Free

Costs of gluten-free foods

One of the main problems with gluten-free foods is their high price. According to a study conducted by the Dalhousie University Medical School the average cost per unit of a product containing gluten is around $0.7, while for a gluten-free product, the average cost per unit is $1.71, the unit being represented, in this study, by 100 grams of product.

While this difference can seem insignificant at first sight, it's actually quite an important aspect if we consider long-term diets, as one eats more than 100 grams of gluten-free bread per week. The same study revealed that, on average, the costs for gluten-free products were 242% higher than the costs for regular foods in the same categories.

Still, this isn't always the case, as celiac disease sufferers and people with intolerance to gluten can avoid this protein without investing huge amounts of money in gluten-free commercial products. A diet that's based on fresh fruits and veggies, lean meat and dairy can be easily kept gluten-free, as the main source of gluten in one's diet is usually represented by grains.

Some simple tips to keep costs at a minimum when eating gluten-free are given below:

- Reducing the intake of junk and processed foods, even if they're labeled "gluten-free". It's a lot healthier and less costly to prepare a dish containing potatoes, chicken and salad at home than to order it from a restaurant or fast food producer that can't always guarantee the products weren't contaminated with gluten.

- Instead of buying gluten-free deserts, eat more fresh fruits, seeds and nuts, as these are naturally free of gluten, have fewer calories and are overall more beneficial for your health state, whether you have gluten sensitivity or not.

- Eat more freshly cooked meat and reduce the intake of processed ones, as even if they shouldn't contain gluten, these products can be contaminated if manipulated with utensils that haven't been thoroughly cleaned. Instead of ordering crispy, prepare your own chicken dish that's gluten-free and healthier.

- Try replacing commercial gluten-free flours with products that are naturally free of gluten, such as almond flour, rice flour or teff flour.

Stocking the kitchen with gluten-free foods

Stocking your kitchen with gluten-free products can be quite costly at the beginning but you can save time and money by creating a list of foods you'll need mostly. These should be the first ones to buy, then depending on your budget and needs, you can continue stocking up the kitchen.

Chances to sticking with the gluten-free diet long enough to actually start seeing improvements in your health are a lot higher if there aren't any gluten-based products in your kitchen. No matter how strong your will is, if you keep biscuits, crackers, bread and other products that do contain gluten in your kitchen, it's quite likely that one day you'll feel tempted to have a gluten-based snack.

So start with this simple change if you want to overcome the temptation of going back to your non GF lifestyle. Given below is a quick list of products that should be in the kitchen of a gluten-free beginner.

For the cooking and baking staple:

- Brown rice, as it's healthier than white rice. Make sure you check the label and choose a producer that's trustworthy, as you don't want the rice to be contaminated with gluten

- Brown rice pasta

- Brown rice flour

- Buckwheat flour, which is gluten-free despite its name

- Quinoa, as it's free of gluten unless cross-contaminated, and it's an excellent source of proteins and fibers. It's tasty and can successfully replace couscous or rice

- Quinoa flakes

- Millet, excellent for gluten-free side dishes

- Millet flour, very food for baking and coating fish or chicken when pan-frying

- Amaranth flour

- Cornstarch, as even if it's a highly refined product, it is sometimes necessary for baking and for thickening dishes. It's a good flour substitute and it's usually less costly than gluten-free flour

- Olive oil

- Canola oil

- Mixtures of beans and legumes, such as white beans, black-eyed peas, kidney beans, pinto beans, split peas, tofu, lentils, chickpeas. These are excellent sources of fibers, proteins and good carbohydrates and they're excellent for vegetarian and vegan dishes. Also, they're free of gluten and the risk of cross-contamination is reduced unless you buy them from bulk bins

- Soy milk

- Soy cheese

- Rice milk

- Chicken stock

- Veggie cooking stock

- Almond cheese

- Mixtures of nuts and seeds, such as walnuts, macadamias, hazelnuts, pistachios, pecans, almonds

- Besides these products, make sure to always have fresh meat and dairy products as well as fresh fruits and vegetables in your kitchen, as the temptation of grabbing a quick, highly processed and unhealthy gluten-based snack decreases drastically when your stomach is full with healthy and nourishing foods.

- And speaking of snacks and the temptation of eating commercial products that contain gluten, coping with cravings is another frequent problem experienced by people who switch to a gluten-free lifestyle.

Coping with cravings when going gluten-free

When first switching to a gluten-free diet, lots of people experience frequent hunger pangs and cravings as their bodies are used to receiving higher amounts of grain and carbohydrates. This is why the best strategy for preventing these cravings for sugar and carbs is to simply replace those grains that contain gluten with gluten-free alternatives.

Then, you should also incorporate more nourishing foods in your menu and increase the intake of proteins and fibers as these are more fulfilling and can keep hunger pangs away. Still, if your cravings are not caused by hunger pangs and are just the result of the gluten addiction that developed in time, here's what you can do to keep them under control:

- Remove all gluten-based products from your diet and search for snacks and deserts that are free of gluten, such as fruit salads, plain yogurts without gluten-based flavors, nuts, seeds, homemade peanut butter or almond butter and other similar products. You can also prepare your own cookies and sweets if you find it too difficult to give up these products, but make sure you use gluten-free ingredients. And keep in mind that nut butters make great replacements for gluten-based sweets!

- Make sure to get enough rest as cravings for sugar are often the result of low energy levels, which are the consequence of restless sleep or lack of sleep. Your body needs 6-8 hours of sleep daily so if you constantly skip rest, you shouldn't be surprised you crave for sweets more often.

- Stay active, as physical activities improve circulation and absorption of nutrients, regulate blood sugar levels and keep your mood elevated. As known, mood swings, depression, increased stress levels and a poor absorption of nutrients can all lead to abnormal cravings for sweets and sugars and unfortunately most of these products are gluten-based. Physical exercises can keep all these under control so you should exercise daily or if you don't have time for complex workouts, try to get at least 60 minutes of jogging or walking every other day the least.

- Avoid stimulants such as cigarettes, alcohol and caffeine. Although some people think these can curb cravings, the truth is they actually increase them due to the effects these products have on the nervous system. Not to mention lots of alcoholic beverages contain gluten so they should be completely removed from your menu.

- Try to spend more time outdoor, as exposure to sunlight and fresh air improves your overall health, making it less likely to experience abnormal cravings for sugars and products containing gluten.

- If these strategies don't work, your body might lack certain nutrients so you should check your mineral and vitamin levels and supplement, if needed, the daily intake of the missing nutrients.

- Some natural supplements can diminish cravings as well: Ginkgo biloba, St. John's wort, acetyl-l-carnitine, vitamin B6 and vitamin B3 derivatives.

Preventing cross-contamination at home

Another common problem with gluten-free diets is that lots of products that are free of gluten can be contaminated even when cooking at home, if you previously used the utensils or dishes for preparing other foods, non GF. Here are some strategies you can apply for avoiding cross-contamination at home:

- Always clean the surfaces after preparing dishes with gluten-based ingredients.

- Make sure your hands and the utensils you're using while cooking are perfectly clean, before and after food preparation. Gluten-free dishes must never be prepared in a floury atmosphere, especially if you're often using wheat flour.

- Use separate utensils for butter, margarine, jam, pickles, bread and other products that might contain gluten. Even the smallest amount of this ingredient can cause unpleasant reactions to gluten intolerant persons.

- When cooking multiple foods, always use separate dishes for gluten-based and gluten-free products.

Gluten-free foods to take with you while traveling

Another very common problem for people going gluten-free is finding some easy to make recipes that can be taken with them while traveling. Lots of people find it stressful to search for restaurants offering gluten-free menus when spending lots of time traveling and carrying foods in a bag for several days is not really recommended, so the best foods for travelers are those that can resist unaltered for more days in a row even in high temperatures. Here are some examples:

- Hard-boiled eggs
- Canned chicken
- Tuna or salmon packets
- String cheese

- Beef jerky
- Cauliflower and broccoli, raw or heated
- Oranges
- Apples
- Bananas
- Avocados
- Pears
- Nectarines
- Tangerines
- Peanut butter
- Dried fruits
- Nuts
- Almonds
- GF protein bars
- Freeze dried food packets
- Cooked rice
- Steamed veggies
- GF crackers

While these can all be carried in the car, keep in mind that traveling by plane has different rules and airline companies may not allow the transportation of such foods with you while flying. It's therefore always recommended to check their terms before preparing your food packs when traveling by plane.